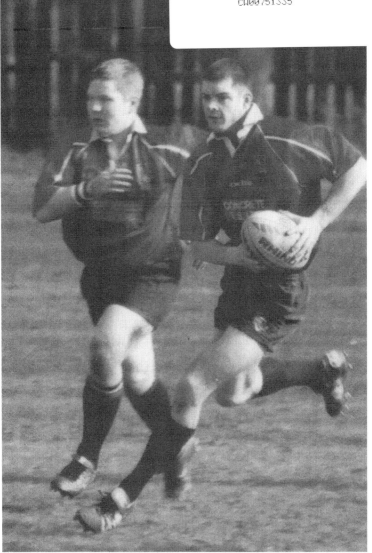

For Dan

When will we see your like again

17 days

The Shocking
True Story of Dan's
Cancer Diagnosis

Anne Logan Huxtable

WORDCATCHER publishing

17 Days
The Shocking True Story of Dan's Cancer Diagnosis

© 2016 Anne Logan Huxtable
© All photographs friends and family, except
p.32 © North West Evening Mail.

British Library Cataloguing in Publication Data.
A catalogue record for this book is available from the British Library.

Published in the United Kingdom by Wordcatcher Publishing
www.wordcatcher.com
Tel: 02921 888321
Facebook.com/WordcatcherPublishing

First Edition: October, 2016
First published by Octavo Publishing Ltd

ISBN: 9781912056996
Second Edition: April 2017

Category: True Stories

Contents

Foreword 1

Prologue...7

CHAPTER 1 15
Friday, 4th April, 2003

Chapter 2 21
Saturday, 5th April 2003 (Midnight)

Chapter 3 29
Sunday, 6th April, 2003

Chapter 4 33
Monday, 7th April, 2003

Chapter 5 37
Tuesday, 8th April, 2003

Chapter 6 43
Wednesday, 9th April, 2003

Chapter 7 49
Thursday, 10th April, 2003 (Midnight)

Chapter 8 53
Friday, 11th April, 2003 (Midnight)

Chapter 9 59
Saturday, 12th April, 2003

Chapter 10 63

    Sunday, 13th April, 2003

Chapter 11 69

    Monday, 14th April, 2003 (Midnight)

Chapter 12 75

    Tuesday, 15th April, 2003

Chapter 13 81

    Wednesday, 16th April, 2003

Chapter 14 89

    Thursday, 17th April, 2003

Chapter 15 101

    Friday, 18th April, 2003

Chapter 16 107

Chapter 17 111

    Tuesday, 29th April, 2003 (1.30pm)

Chapter 18 119

    Events

Aftermath 123

Epilogue 127

Acknowledgements 137

Foreword

Speaking as a father of two, I can't comprehend how I could possibly love my children more than I do; I can only describe it as a feeling so overwhelming that it is joyous yet painful at the same time. But I do believe it is possible and only by a mother. Call it love, a bond or even an extra-sensory perception, I don't know for sure, but I believe it is more than love because the mother has nurtured, carried and been physically connected to the unborn child for nearly 10 months; that is an amazing journey for both.

Less of my ramblings regarding parents and children and on to my good friend Dan. Truly, words are not enough to describe this lad and the saying 'seeing is believing' fit perfectly here but I will try and do him justice…

I met Dan through Vickers Rugby Union Football Club (VRUFC). The environment was typical rugby club but with the emphasis on inclusion and looking out for each other. Nights out could be rowdy but we never caused trouble, no mean feat when there was usually 15-20+ of us on an average night.

There were no formal introductions but Dan and I just gravitated towards each other. This was unlikely given that I was the club's social secretary (non-player, professional drinker and general entertainment) while Dan was tall, physically fit, laid back and quietly confident. Well, they do say opposites attract.

The nights out started with post-match drinks to wash down the infamous club pie and peas, then multiple taxis to the Steelworks pub for karaoke. To my recollection, Dan never got on the mic but he and the lads always sang along, then broke into choruses of our own club songs; much to the disgust of the local rugby league lads! Singing in a group is very much part of our rugby club, it somehow binds the group together, it's like a tribal instinct and it always felt good.

Then followed the 'Gaza Strip Run' (probably not PC to call it that); a run of pubs, bars and clubs on Cornwallis Street, where the real partying took place. This was the birthplace of the 'Breezer Challenge', which involved a bottle of alcopop and a bendy straw – this enabled the drink to be consumed in approximately three seconds. Let's just say where Dan excelled in athleticism I made up for in drinking prowess; but he always competed.

A regular event on the rugby social calendar was a cross-dressing pub crawl. One event (Bez's birthday), was themed on Harry Enfield's Young Man. Thirty young men dressed as older ladies, oh, and it was a bike ride. Most of the lads had trawled Barrow's charity shops for their outfits; though some were slender enough to fit into their girlfriends' clothes (so they said). Dan had gone down the charity shop route and looked a treat – he'd even gone to the trouble of finding a lipstick to match his handbag.

Truly great memories, but Dan was off to university so the nights out weren't as frequent but still as good when we got together. I miss those times…

So, back to where I started on this foreword, and the relationship between a parent and child. I can't really explain it but the story told in the following pages will give an insight into this unbreakable bond.

As I mentioned I am now a father. On 26th November 2009 mine and Hayley's first child was born, a son, six weeks premature and fighting after a traumatic birth. He's now six and a strapping young boy. We named him Logan...

To Dan, from all of the lads:

We're all going up to Sunshine
Mountain, faces all aglow – oh-oh-oh.
Turn around you warrior and reach up
to the sky.
We're all going up to Sunshine
Mountain, you and I...

Martin Sainty

Prologue

Daniel William weighed in at 7lbs 2ozs on Thursday, 18th December 1980, at Risedale Maternity Hospital in Barrow-in- Furness. He was a long, slim baby with dark hair and beautiful, almond-shaped, brown eyes.

My marriage to Dan's father broke up when Dan was six months old, and for a few years I was a single parent. The bond between us was strong – it was the two of us.

Dan was a lovely-natured, affectionate little boy. He was strong-willed; once his mind was made up there was no turning back – that led to the occasional tantrum; especially in Marks and Spencer, where he would drop on his back like a starfish.

In 1986 I remarried, Dan wanted his surname changed to Logan to be the same as my husband George, and myself.

He enjoyed his years at Newbarns Infant and Junior schools, he loved being involved in activities. Aged nine, he was awarded the Cub of the Year Trophy at St. Aidan's Scout Group.

From the age of eleven, Dan attended Thorncliffe School, (now sadly demolished). The school excelled at basketball, which became his first love. Dan was thrilled at his first training session when his coach, Ian France, realised Dan was left-handed and gave him a special set of moves to practice. He played for the Cadet and Junior teams, where he was two years younger than his teammates, and captained the Junior team when he was 16. His kit wasn't complete without his 'lucky' socks – white with a green Nike swoosh! I was his biggest fan. Along with other mums, I travelled around the country in a minibus supporting the team.

Dan gained refereeing and coaching qualifications and helped run summer basketball camps.

For a couple of seasons, he also played football for a local team – I spent many Saturdays standing on touchlines in the wind and rain.

Dan gained six GCSEs and received the Physical Education Prize, along with the Annual Gold Award for Sporting Achievements at Thorncliffe School's award ceremony in December 1997. He went on to study Sociology, IT, and Sports Studies at

Barrow Sixth Form College.

Probably because he was an only child, Dan was mature for his age and gravitated towards an older age group for friends. He was friendly and easygoing but didn't suffer fools gladly.

One evening, a mate invited him to a training session at Vickers Rugby Union Club – he was immediately hooked and signed on as a winger.

I said "Are you mad? You'll get flattened!"

He was indeed bruised and battered after his first game, but he said, "I loved it, it was brilliant!"

When I grumbled about washing his muddy kit, he'd say, "Stop your whingeing, woman," then he'd grin and add, "Thanks Mam."

Vickers' coach Jeff Simm took Dan under his wing and became his mentor. Despite the age difference they became good mates. The lads joked that Dan had been adopted by Jeff; a lovely man, sadly no longer with us.

Dan worked out and trained hard to progress to the first team. He was described as a 'pacy' winger. He loved rugby, the team ethos, and, of course, the social events.

Dan gave 100% to everything he did, whether it was work, sport, or having a good time.

The bond between us grew stronger over the years. We shared the same attitude to life, and supported and advised each other when one of us had a problem.

On the rare occasions Dan had a free Saturday, he'd say, "Are you going to town? I'll come with you. We'll have a cuppa and a catch-up." Like his mother, Dan was a tea addict.

Dan had a great sense of humour. His favourite comedian was Peter Kay and he'd often text me one liners – "It's that fine rain, Mother," or, "It's the future, Jerry."

Dan was bitterly disappointed he didn't achieve the A-level results he required and he re-sat the exams in 2000. We rose early on the morning the results were due. Someone had made an error – the letter, offering him a place at Edge Hill University in Ormskirk, arrived before he'd collected his results from Sixth Form! We hugged each other and danced around the kitchen.

"Oh Dan, I'm so proud of you. I'm so

happy for you."

I was thinking, *He's going away. What will I do without him. I'll miss him so much.*

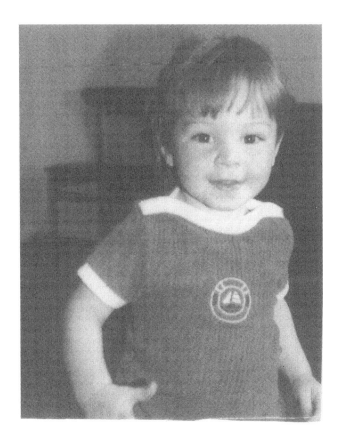

The safety gate was in place at the top of the stairs so that toddler Daniel could play upstairs while I had a quick bath. Several times I asked him, "What are you playing with Daniel?"

"Colours."

I came out of the bathroom to find he'd unscrewed the top from a bottle of nail polish and painted the lens of my glasses bright orange!

CHAPTER 1

Friday, 4th April, 2003

I shivered, not entirely due to the early morning chill, as I waited for the 8.25am train at Barrow in Furness. I was going to see my son, Dan, who was a third-year student at Edge Hill University in Ormskirk, Lancashire.

He'd sent a text the previous evening –
Been in hospital for 3 hours this afternoon.

I'd phoned him immediately, and he told me, "I had awful stomach pains and I'm being sick so I went to the A&E Department. They think it's a stomach infection and I've got antibiotics – they're like horse pills, Mam."

Dan had been nauseous for a few days. Initially we put this down to a riotous weekend in Liverpool with the rugby team, but when he didn't feel better after 24 hours we thought perhaps he had a virus. My concern heightened when he added, "I'm not going to Belgium on Saturday – I feel too rough." He had been looking forward to the University rugby team tour for weeks. I knew he really was ill if he was foregoing that trip.

"I think you need some TLC from your Mam. I'll come down tomorrow on the train."

He didn't argue.

I arrived at the three-storey house in Knowsley Road late morning and went straight to Dan's attic room (a.k.a. 'The Penthouse'). He was in bed, really pale, and dark shadows under his eyes. I hugged him.

"How are you feeling, mate?"

"Rough. I took a tablet earlier but I've been sick since then."

I freshened him up and made him a drink. He hadn't eaten since the previous day. I suggested something plain to put a lining on his stomach. I walked the short distance to the town centre and bought myself a pie and tinned custard for Dan. He ate a small amount, but vomited without warning soon afterwards. He was weak; I had to help him from the bed to the chair so I could change the sheets.

While Dan drifted in and out of sleep, I dug out his sleeping bag and cleared some floor space. His housemate, Helen, came to see how he was. She offered me her room, which was next to Dan's, as her (then) partner Mark also had a room in the house and she could stay with him. She made the bed up for me and brought me a cup of tea; a lovely, caring young woman.

When Dan woke up he had stomach pains. I gave him the antibiotic that was due; he vomited a few minutes later. I was prepared and had tissues and a bucket ready. Dan's mate, Sion, who shared the house and played rugby with Dan, came up to see how he was. His contribution was, "I'll have your share of beer in Belgium!"

Dan dozed for a while, then we watched Top of the Pops. To this day, if I hear Simply Red singing *Sunrise* I'm transported back to that room.

I gave Dan the last antibiotic of the day at 10pm and made him comfortable.

***

"What are you doing?" I screeched as I stumbled, bleary eyed, into the kitchen one morning and saw ten-year old Dan pouring water from the previous night's hot water bottle into the kettle.

"I'm saving water. We've talked about it at school. You mustn't waste the Earth's resources." Apparently, he'd made me a cup of tea every morning that week using recycled water...

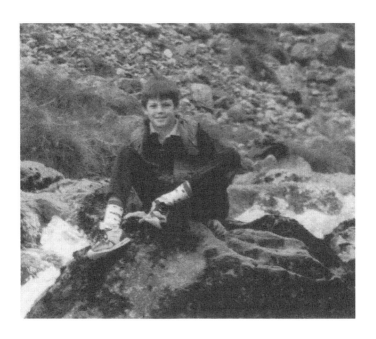

Chapter 2

Saturday, 5th April 2003
(Midnight)

I went in to Dan several times during the night. He vomited thick, brown liquid: I felt ill looking at it. The infection wouldn't clear up if he couldn't keep the tablets in his system. He had also developed a harsh cough. There was no doubt he needed to see a doctor.

I rushed downstairs to the lounge and rummaged through the cupboards for a phone book, only to wake Sion's brother, who was sleeping on the sofa. I don't know which of us was more startled.

I phoned GP surgeries, but all I heard were recorded messages saying they were closed on Saturday. Thankfully, the last number was answered. When I explained the situation, the receptionist transferred me to a GP. He asked a few questions, then said, "My concern is dehydration. Rather than wait for me to make a house call, I'd advise that he goes to hospital. You can take him yourself or I can arrange for an ambulance."

My stomach lurched.

"I'll take him. Thank you."

At the best of times, I don't function well without a cup of tea; at that moment, I was in a panic.

I made a drink and ran upstairs, yelling, "Whose car is blocking Dan's?"

Sion opened her door, said 'Martin', and pointed to another door.

I banged on Martin's door. "Move your car, please. I have to take Dan to hospital."

I quickly washed and dressed and went to Dan. "I'm sorry mate, but you have to go to hospital." He pulled a face, then doubled over in pain, holding his stomach. I helped him to dress and put his trainers on. I guided him down the stairs one at a time. I was scared he would lose his balance and fall down three flights of stairs. The lads stood around on the landing.

"Bloody hell, Dan! You look like shite!"

"I feel like shite."

I helped Dan into the car and he directed me to Ormskirk General Hospital, a few minutes' drive away. It was 8.30am.

We were soon called to the treatment area. Dr Suma, who had treated Dan 48 hours earlier, was on duty. He said "I thought you were pale then, but you're even paler now."

All the cubicles were occupied, so Dan had to lie on a trolley in the corridor. Dr Suma told us the dark-coloured vomit (known as coffee grounds) was digested blood. He said "I know you're a student and you like to have a good time, but have you been binge drinking?"

"No."

When Dr Suma walked away, I said sharply, "Have you? Tell me."

"No. I haven't, honestly."

I believed him.

A nurse set up a saline drip and took blood samples. Dr Suma returned and gave Dan a pain-killing injection. He said "You need a blood transfusion. I think you have a bleeding stomach ulcer. I want to admit you for some tests. I'm trying to find a bed for you."

We were stunned.

The only time Dan had been in hospital was when he was born. He said "I'm glad you're here, Mam. I couldn't do this on my own."

I took hold of his hand, "Hey, I'm your Mam. I'll always be here."

I turned away so he wouldn't see the tears in my eyes. He was 22 but he was still my little lad.

Dan was a strong, active young man. He played rugby for Edge Hill and Liverpool St Helens. He was studying Sports Science. His plan was to join the RAF as a physical training instructor. His diet was healthy. What could have caused an ulcer?

I said "I need a brew. I'll only be a minute." I stood by the vending machine and took deep breaths.

Time passed slowly. A bed became available late in the afternoon. Dan was settled in a small room at the end of Ward F, which was a female medical ward.

A nurse set up the blood transfusion.

I told Dan "I'll collect your toiletries and stuff and I'll be right back." It was 5pm and I had to leave anyway as it was dinner time.

At the car, I realised I had no idea how to get back to Knowsley Road. I asked at reception for directions; I must have driven to the hospital on autopilot that morning.

The student house was empty. Most of the housemates had gone home for the Easter holidays. I scribbled a note saying Dan was having blood transfusions and stuck it to the banister rail.

I checked his toiletries, then walked to the

town centre for a few extra items. The sun was shining. It was unseasonably warm and I had packed jeans and jumpers in my overnight bag. I hastily purchased a cotton blouse.

Helen and Mark were home when I got back to the house. They were shocked that Dan was in hospital. Helen hugged me and sent Mark to make me a cup of tea. I phoned my husband, George, to bring him up to date, and let Dan's best mate, Dan Jones (Jonesy), who lived locally, know that Dan hadn't gone to Belgium.

Dan was sat up when I went back to the hospital at 6pm. He said "I feel a bit better now. How long do you think I'll have to stay here?"

"A couple of days, probably. Then we'll get you home and I'll look after you."

"Sounds good."

A nurse checked him and set up another unit of blood.

I bought a payment card for the TV and we watched a repeat of the Grand National and chatted. I was queasy with hunger: all I had eaten that day was a chocolate biscuit from the vending machine.

"Which takeaway do you use?"

"Go to Pacino's. That's the best."

I kissed Dan goodnight.

"See you tomorrow. Phone me if you want anything."

He settled down to read his Andy McNab novel.

I parked the car and walked into the town centre again. The evening was still warm. The streets were full of young people in their Saturday night finery. It felt surreal. *What am I doing here?*

I walked up and down looking for Pacino's. Eventually, I bought a bag of chips from the Marmaris.

I phoned George and we arranged for him to come to Ormskirk the next day. I gave him a list of clothes to bring. I would be staying longer than just the weekend. I moved my belongings from Helen's room to Dan's and wearily fell into bed.

"I made 50p on the pie run today!"

Dan was a fast runner. His schoolmates gave him their money at lunchtime and he ran to the nearby bakery for pies. They didn't have to queue and Dan got to keep the change – it was a win-win situation

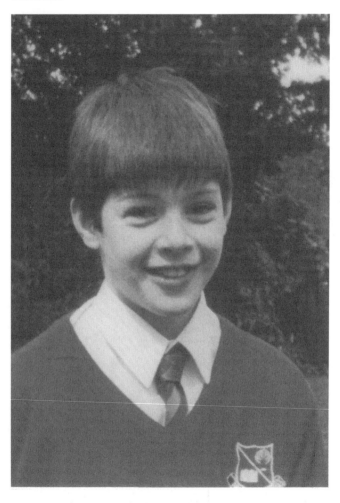

Chapter 3

Sunday, 6th April, 2003

I slept very little. I couldn't believe Dan was in hospital. I woke for the umpteenth time and saw a note had been pushed under the door. It was from Martin, inviting me to have breakfast at Slim Jim's Jazz Cafe, which he managed. I gathered up all my courage and braved the student shower room. The less said about that, the better!

I walked through town for the third time in 16 hours. Again, the weather was warm and sunny. I brought Martin up to date and enjoyed a full English breakfast on the house! On the way back through town I bought food and wine, then spent the rest of the morning cleaning the kitchen and threatening students with violence it they didn't keep it clean.

George arrived at lunchtime, my Dad had accompanied him. When we visited at 2pm, Dan was having a further blood transfusion. His face had lost the pallor of the previous day. He said "I've eaten breakfast and lunch. I feel a lot better."

During evening visiting, Jonesy, Stuart Carter, and their girlfriends visited. They thought it was hilarious that I was living in the student house. I said "I wandered around for ages last night looking for Pacino's. I couldn't find it so I went to the Marmaris." They all sniggered.

Dan said "Ah. That is Pacino's. They changed the name!"

"Oh nice one, son."

I stayed with Dan till 9pm. I was confident he would be discharged the next day.

Back at the house, I made a sandwich, poured a glass of wine and lay on Dan's bed watching his British Lions video, *Up Close and Personal with the Lions.* I thought I could do this. I could be a student!

* * *

Dan, aged 16, playing for Thorns Basketball Club.

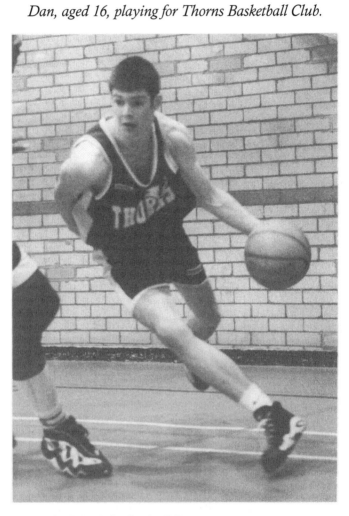

Picture Credit: North West Evening Mail

Chapter 4

Monday, 7th April, 2003

I phoned Ward F at 8am and was told Dan had spent a comfortable night. I gathered together two bags of clothes and bedding and spent the morning in the local launderette. I bought some Complan for Dan, thinking it was easy to digest and wouldn't aggravate his stomach.

My Mam travelled by train that day to see Dan. We had lunch in town, then I drove us to the hospital.

I was taken aback when I saw Dan. He was pale; he'd vomited a couple of times that morning and didn't want to eat. I found a nurse, who told me Dan was scheduled to have a gastroscopy on Thursday. I couldn't understand why he had to wait so long when he was already an in-patient.

During evening visiting, Jonesy and his dad, Bob, called in, along with Christan Upton, another mate and rugby player. They didn't stay long, they could see Dan wasn't up to talking much.

"What time are you leaving?" Dan asked me.

"I can go now, if you're tired?"

"No, don't go. I don't want to be on my own."

"I'll stay as long as you want then." Dan needed to use the bathroom. He was unsteady on his feet, so I supported him. His faeces were black and tarry due to the digested blood passing through his system. I cleaned him, then made him comfortable in bed.

I asked him, "Do you think I'd make a good nurse?"

"Yeah, you're not doing bad!"

He was asleep when I left at 10.30pm.

"Oh navy blue and pearls, you can't go wrong son," *I said, as Dan sashayed into the living room.*

George spluttered "Don't flamin' encourage him!"

Dan was wearing a flowered calf- length dress, navy floppy hat and a string of pearls.

Rugby mate Simon Rodgers was celebrating his birthday and he'd decreed the lads should go on a pub crawl while riding bikes and dressed as women.

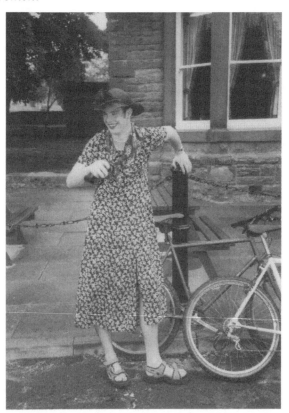

Chapter 5

Tuesday, 8th April, 2003

I had another uneasy night. I phoned Ward F and was told Dan was comfortable.

He was asleep when I visited at 2pm. I'd bought a big 'Get Well' balloon that morning and I weighted it in the corner of his room. He laughed when he saw it. "I'm twenty-two!"

"It was that or flowers! Anyway, how are you feeling?"

"I've been for an x-ray 'cos I'm coughing, but it's alright."

The truth was, the radiographer had said 'That's alright', meaning 'The x-ray has been taken successfully'. Dan had never had an x-ray, so he assumed she was referring to the results.

I smelt the staleness of his body and his breath as I leaned over to kiss his cheek. "I'm not being funny mate, but you need a shower."

"I know, I'd love one. I tried to get out of bed this morning but I was dizzy. The walls were spinning."

I looked at him. "Shall we do it between us? I'm not embarrassed if you're not."

"Let's do it."

I gathered his toiletries and helped him sit up on the edge of the bed. He stood and leaned against me. At 6' 4", he towered over me. I supported him around the waist, and he put his arm around my shoulder. Slowly, we walked the few steps across the corridor to the shower room. He half-fell onto the plastic chair: his weight was too much for me.

Dan's face was drained of colour. I shampooed and rinsed his hair; then soaped up the facecloth and washed his back, chest, and arms. The scent of Lynx Africa filled the room. I soaped the cloth again and handed it to him.

"Here – you can do your own bits, I'm not doing those!"

He managed a smile.

I rinsed the suds off and gently dried him with his Scotland rugby towel. I knelt and guided his feet into clean boxer shorts. He leaned on me to rise from the chair and I pulled the shorts over his hips. Again, with his arm around my shoulder, I supported him and we slowly shuffled back to his room. He was exhausted.

Back at the house I made a sandwich, but I couldn't swallow it, my throat felt closed. I started crying. Dan was weaker now than when he was admitted. Still vomiting and coughing up frothy sputum, he definitely wasn't improving.

When I went back at 6pm, Dan's untouched meal was on the table. He said "I don't want it. I feel sick."

I had taken yoghurt in with me, he ate a few teaspoonfuls but violently vomited coffee grounds a short while later. I cleaned him up and disposed of the bowl in the sluice room. I supported him while he urinated into a vessel; he didn't have the strength to stand up. I washed him, washed my hands, disposed of the vessel, then washed my hands again. I was scared he would catch MRSA.

I stayed with Dan till late, then kissed him goodnight: "See you tomorrow. I love you."

"I love you Mam."

As I reached the doorway he asked, "Will you record 'The Sopranos' for me? I don't want to miss any."

* * *

"Hiya Mam, I'm having the best weekend of my life." Dan could hardly speak at 9am one Saturday.

"You sound rough."

"We were drinking with some Americans till 5 o'clock this morning."

Dan and 41 mates from Vickers Rugby Club had gone to Twickenham for the cup final, dressed as Elvis. They walked from the tube station up to the overland platform, wearing white jumpsuits and rubber mask quiffs. The station announcer said, "Ladies and Gentlemen, Elvis has entered the station!"

The lads waved graciously as fellow travellers applauded. Dan saw his hero Lawrence Dallaglio play, and Wasps won the final. A weekend fit for The King!

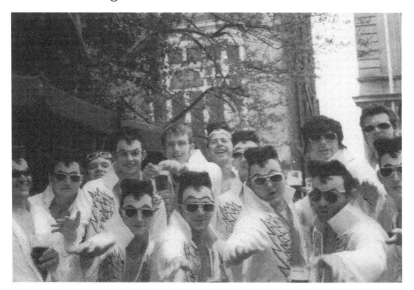

Chapter 6

Wednesday, 9th April, 2003

I was told Dan had spent a comfortable night when I phoned the ward.

I went shopping for soft food to tempt him. I hoped that if he could eat he would have the strength to fight off whatever illness he had.

When I went in at 2pm, he was lying down. He told me he'd vomited a few times and his stomach was 'off colour'. He asked "Can I have a shower again?"

We repeated the previous day's experience and I had just made him comfortable in bed when Bob Jones came in. Then Dr Suma knocked. He asked to speak to Dan alone.

A couple of minutes later, Dr Suma came out and said, "You can go in now. I'll speak to you soon."

Dan was lying on his side, his face turned to the pillow. I sat on the bed and took his hand. "What is it love? What did he say?"

Dan turned to me, his eyes were brimming with tears. "He thinks I might have cancer."

"NO. NO. I'm not having that."

Bob touched my arm and left. Dr Suma came in. "The x-rays have shown shadows on Dan's lungs. I've arranged scans for Friday; we will know more then.

He is aware of cancer, he told me he has a friend who has it?"

I could only nod. Dan's friend, David Cole, had been diagnosed with testicular cancer three years previously, and was still undergoing treatment. David was two years older than Dan. They had both attended Thorncliffe School and Barrow Sixth Form College, where they had both played basketball for the school and college teams.

Two sports-mad, healthy young men. Two only children.

Two December birthdays.

The similarities were uncanny.

I sat on Dan's bed and we gripped each other's hands. Neither of us spoke. Thoughts whirled around in my head. *Maybe he has Tuberculosis.* I knew there had been a resurgence of the disease in recent years. *That's curable. He's had the vaccinations at school. He can take time off uni. He'll be alright.*

Dan broke the silence. "Do you want to phone George?"

"He won't be home yet." We sat holding hands.

At 5.30pm I said, "I'll be as quick as I can." Dan nodded.

I leaned against the wall in the lift. I was dazed. My hands shook so much that I struggled to unlock the car. I slumped over the steering wheel and sobbed, "Not my Dan. Please, not my Dan."

When George answered the phone, I managed to gasp, "It's me."

"What is it? What's wrong?" "They think Dan has cancer." "My god, no."

I told him what Dr Suma had said. "I'll be with you as soon as I can."

I composed myself and went back to Dan. I pulled the chair up next to the bed and held his hand. A nurse came in to take his temperature. I told her "I'm staying here tonight. I'm not leaving him on his own."

I expected some opposition, but she replied, "I'll bring you some blankets." She added "I can get you an armchair with a footrest. You'll be more comfortable."

I thanked her.

Dan spluttered and began to vomit. I supported his weight while he was sick and cleaned him up. Then he needed to urinate. Again, I held him, washed him, then disposed of the vessels.

George arrived at about 8.30pm. I leaned against him. He was shocked at the change in Dan in the three short days since he had seen him.

We whispered while Dan slept. Neither of us could take in what was happening. Dan woke abruptly and vomited coffee grounds. I cleaned him up and disposed of the bowl.

I asked George "Who's looking after Jake?" (Our family cat).

"Nobody. I just left him." Dan snorted.

'Jakesie Cat', as Dan called him, was a handsome, affectionate tuxedo cat. He used to stretch out with his paws facing upwards. Dan was convinced Jake was gay.

Later in the evening I curled up in the armchair next to the bed while George sat in the corner.

Jake Edge, Dan's other persona, was born on an Edge Hill rugby tour to Edinburgh. Jake wore the Saltire around his shoulders and a pair of blue rubber gloves, (the gloves were a punishment from the kangaroo court for washing dishes in the student house).

Jake was the saviour of the world. He was an awesome character and apparently offered the coach driver a lap dance on the way back to Edge Hill.

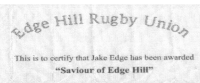

Edge Hill Rugby Union

This is to certify that Jake Edge has been awarded
"Saviour of Edge Hill"

Thank you Jake for your continued Service to the
World and Edge Hill

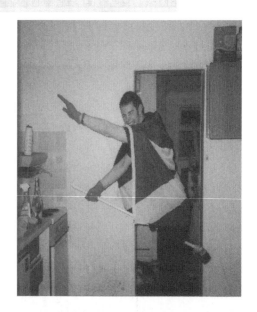

Chapter 7

Thursday, 10th April, 2003
(Midnight)

Dan had a bad night. He vomited several times and needed to urinate frequently. He was stressed: "What's wrong with me? Why am I like this?"

"I'm not sure sweetheart. We have to wait for the tests."

I felt helpless.

Dan was even weaker and couldn't stand unaided. A shower was out of the question. I washed him, and he let George shave him. Dan sipped some water but refused to eat anything.

Mid-morning, a porter came to take Dan for a pelvic scan. I managed to pull a t-shirt over Dan's head, and we helped him into the wheelchair. He slumped forward, not having the strength to sit upright.

George and I waited outside the x-ray department. Dan looked terrible when the porter wheeled him out. Back in his room, we had to lift him onto the bed.

Later, we were told the pelvic scan was clear. I felt relief to a small extent. At least he doesn't have *that*.

During the afternoon, a different porter

came to take Dan for the gastroscopy. I insisted he was wheeled to the theatre in his bed: "He almost passed out this morning; he's not getting in that chair."

Dan was extremely distressed after the procedure. "I was choking. I wanted to be sick. It was awful. Don't let them do that to me again, Mam. Promise."

I promised him. The gastroscopy revealed an acute gastric ulcer.

During the week, Dan's housemates and rugby mates called in regularly; they were shocked at his appearance. They only stayed a few minutes, they could see he wasn't up to visitors.

Dan's friend, a lovely young girl called Kerry Medcalf, visited along with her friend. Dan was drifting in and out of sleep, Kerry was upset when she saw how ill he looked.

Jonesy's Mum, Jackie, visited that evening. She brought a platter of sandwiches and savouries and continued to do so every day we were in Ormskirk Hospital. She was a huge support to us. She also brought a dish of jelly for Dan. I fed him a few teaspoonfuls of 'Mrs Jones's Magic Jelly', as it became known.

* * *

"Mam, do you fancy going to Murrayfield to see Scotland and The All Blacks? I can get cheap tickets 'cos I'm a student."

"I'd love to, but wouldn't you rather go with your mates?"

"They're all busy that Saturday, I thought you and me could go."

The atmosphere at Murrayfield was amazing; pipe bands, military displays and fireworks, plus the Haka. I was surprised that Dan knew the words of 'Flower of Scotland.'

"We had to learn it for the Edinburgh tour," *he explained.*

I paid for the tickets and petrol, bought the lunches, the programmes, the goodies in the souvenir store – it was the most expensive cheap day out I'd ever had!

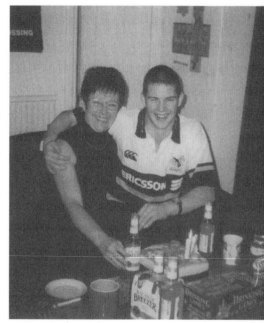

Chapter 8

Friday, 11th April, 2003
(Midnight)

The early hours passed in a cycle of Dan vomiting and needing to urinate. He only passed a few drops of urine at a time.

He said "I'm cold." We added extra blankets, but he asked for his duvet from the house.

I washed him and tried to clean his teeth, which wasn't easy when he was lying down. He didn't want George to shave him: "No. Leave it."

Around 8.30am, I drove to the house to pick up Dan's duvet. While I was in his room, there was a knock on the door. I was stunned to see my brother, Mike. He had driven through the night from his home in Sussex. He said "I had a feeling you needed me."

Dan was surprised to see Uncle Mike when we arrived at the hospital together. Mike said "I thought I'd come and check up on you!"

Mid-morning, Dan was taken for CT scans on his abdomen and chest. Dr Horsley, a Consultant Physician, had arranged to speak to us at 6pm to discuss the results.

Dan continued vomiting and coughing. His sputum was flecked with blood.

During the afternoon, arrangements were made for Dan to have a brain scan. My stomach lurched. *They suspect a brain tumour. Please, no.*

George became agitated at this development; Mike took him outside for some air.

My knees literally knocked together as I sat outside the x-ray department. I knew it was bad news as the porter and a nurse wheeled Dan out: the nurse was wiping tears from her eyes. I started crying, she put her arm around me and walked with me to Dan's room. He had slept all the time.

I sat inbetween George and Mike, opposite Dr Horsley in the day room. He said "I'm afraid it's very bad news. The scans show Daniel has tumours throughout his body. There are too many lung tumours to count. He has a tumour in his heart cavity, which is very rare, and there are two brain tumours. There is nothing we can do. I am very, very sorry."

I burst into tears. Mike put his arm around me, and George and I held hands.

Dr Horsley continued: "We can't locate

the primary site of the cancer and it's futile to treat the secondary sites. I'll start him on steroids and we'll set up a syringe driver to deliver morphine. If Daniel's heart stops, I won't attempt resuscitation: it isn't fair on him, or you."

He explained that the gastric ulcer, which ironically was healing, was caused by the stress of fighting the tumours.

I went onto autopilot. "Are we talking a couple of weeks? A couple of months? What time scale are we talking about?"

"I'm sorry, I don't know."

I discussed palliative care with Dr Horsley. "Can Dan be moved back to Barrow? I want to look after him at home." "It's too far for him to travel. I'll make enquiries about hospices locally."

We left the day-room and stood in Dan's doorway. He was asleep. Mike spoke first "I'll go to Barrow tonight and tell our parents. We can't tell them this on the phone."

My practical voice said, "Will you ask Mam to look after Jake?" I made a list of clothes for Mike to bring back for us. We didn't know where we would be going next. George and I sat in silence. My mind was in turmoil.

There must be a mistake. How can this be happening to my Dan? How can my gorgeous, strong lad have this filthy disease?

A nurse set up the syringe driver, then brought us tea. "You're welcome to use our kitchen to make drinks. There's a side room with a couch, you can try and get some sleep in there." I wouldn't leave Dan so George went to the room.

* * *

"Turn it down" I yelled from the hall, as 'Wonderwall' reverberated through the house on Saturday lunchtime. Dan appeared on the landing.

"Did you know the British Lions played 'Wonderwall' on their tour?"

"No. I didn't."

"Yeah, they got psyched up to it. That's what I'm doing." He flexed his muscles. "I'm getting psyched up for today's game. I'll smash 'em."

"Can you psych up a bit quieter then?"

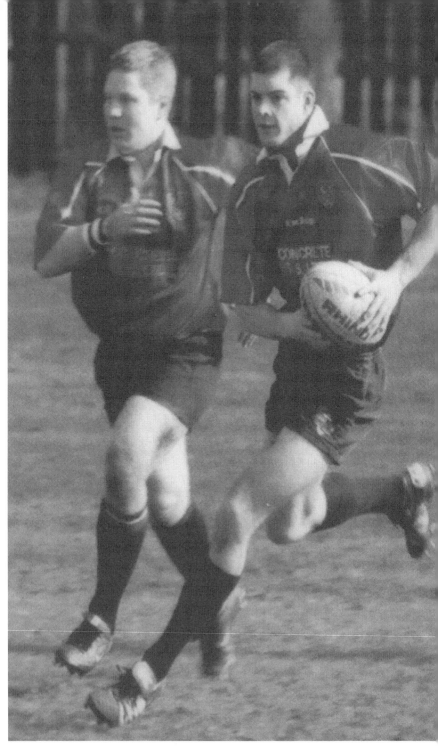

Chapter 9

Saturday, 12th April, 2003

Around 2am I was curled up in the armchair next to Dan, his back was towards me.

He spluttered, then projectile vomited. He couldn't lift his head. He was choking. I ran around the bed and somehow got my arms under his shoulders to lift him. He threw up coffee grounds on me, the bed, the floor and the window blind. It was as if his insides were coming out. I thought This is it. He's dying. This is the end, now.

I managed to stretch across the bed and push the buzzer while still holding him. He had stopped being sick but I couldn't lay him down on the sodden bed. I held him against me.

A nurse came in and exclaimed, "Oh no!" Between us, we stripped the sheets off, while supporting Dan, washed him, sponged the mattress, and made up the bed. I used the basin in his room to get washed and threw my T-shirt in the bin. Tears poured down my face. The nurse brought me tea, but my hands shook so much I could hardly hold the cup. I held Dan's hand while he slept. I was in a nightmare. But

I was awake.

Mike arrived back at the hospital mid-morning. Our parents were obviously devastated – my Dad had said, 'It should be me. Not Dan. I'm old. I've had my life.'

Dan slept during the afternoon and seemed more comfortable, so I left George and Mike in charge while I went to the house for a shower. I worked hard at keeping up a front when I was with Dan, but as soon as I was away from him I fell apart. A combination of fatigue and emotion hit me as I stumbled along the hospital corridor. Tears blinded me as I leaned against the wall in the lift.

The other occupant was an elderly man. He was concerned. "Are you alright, dear?"

I shook my head sobbing, "My son's got cancer. He's dying."

He touched my arm. "I'm sorry."

Mike's wife, Sam, arrived at the hospital. Her father, Chris, had driven her from Sussex.

Paul Carter (father of Dan's friends Dominic and Stuart) came to see how Dan was. He kindly offered Mike and Sam the use of his home, as the family were going away.

Dan's friends were phoning and texting, asking when they could visit. I went onto autopilot once more.

"It's bad news. Dan's had loads of tests, he's got cancer. It's terminal."

They were shocked beyond words. There were many tears.

* * *

Edge Hill rugby tour in Belgium, 2002

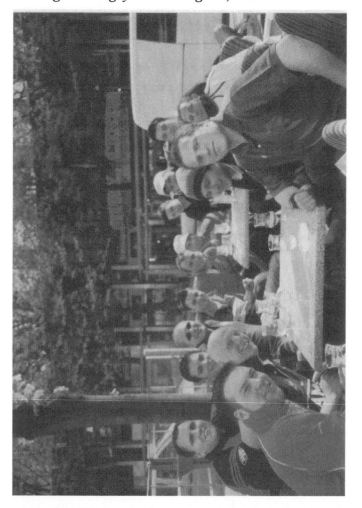

Chapter 10

Sunday, 13th April, 2003

During the early hours, Dan needed to use the commode. I manoeuvred his legs off the bed, but as I helped him to sit up his arm gave way and he fell backwards. He cried out "What's wrong with me? Why can't I sit up?"

"I'm not sure love."

I didn't know what to say. I cleaned him, then manhandled him back into bed. Any movement exhausted him and he slept again. A nurse came in to check his temperature, which was raised. She didn't approve of him being wrapped in his double duvet and brought a table fan, which Dan wanted turned off as soon as she left the room. I queried his arm weakness with her. She replied "His arm will be sore where he's had injections."

I settled down in the armchair again, but a few minutes later Dan vomited coffee grounds. I wiped his face, gave him a sip of water, then disposed of the bowl. I wrapped a blanket around myself, curled up in the chair and closed my eyes.

"MAM. I need a pee." "You're such a charmer."

George came into Dan's room around 6am so that I could try to get some sleep. Dan was restless. I freshened him up and gave him some water. He was agitated and began to cry out. I tried to soothe him while George went for a nurse.

"Where's the pain?" I asked. "My head. I can't stand it."

After a consultation, he was given a pain-killing injection. He was asleep within a minute. The nurse said "I think that was partly stress: the injection usually takes a few minutes to work on pain."

Mike and Sam arrived and, together with George, they pressured me to get some sleep. I was reluctant to leave Dan but they were right; I was light-headed and shaky. I made them promise to phone me if Dan's condition changed. Sam drove me to the house and I slept for a couple of hours.

Dan was just waking when we arrived back at the hospital. I asked "How are you feeling, mate? Any pain anywhere?"

"No."

"That's good. Try to sleep again, you might feel a bit stronger."

"I will when you tell me what's wrong

with me," he answered, in an extremely bolshy tone.

I was caught off-guard. We looked at each other. My son deserved to know the truth. I held his hand and took a deep breath. "The tests show that you have a type of lung cancer. A bit like Coley. The doctors are deciding how to treat it. We're all here and we're going to get you better. We're going to look after you and get you better."

He nodded then closed his eyes. He slept almost straight away. The truth was better than uncertainty.

Mike put his arm around me and said, "That was the bravest thing I've ever seen." During the afternoon Dan Jones and Sion visited. We sat in the corridor and left them with Dan. They were arguing between themselves about a rugby venue at which point Dan managed to speak and put them right!

I walked with them to the car park. We stood with our arms around each other, all of us crying.

Later, my dad arrived, together with his sister and brother-in-law. They all spent time with Dan. Everyone was distressed at seeing him so ill.

* * *

A quote from former prop forward for Vickers Rugby Club, Jason Meadows (known to one and all as 'Big Jase').

"*Can't remember the club, but we'd played rugby and a night out in Blackpool. After a few lemonades, Lionel Ritchie's* Dancing on the Ceiling *came on. Well, it was too much of an invitation. I picked Dan up, upside down, he put his feet on the ceiling and started to dance, much to the annoyance of the bouncers; but with 25 rugby lads in tow they didn't have a say in it.*

"*Once Dan decided he was about to pass out due to the effects of lemonade and the rush of blood to his head, we lowered the lad back down to terra firma. Great night, great memories.*"

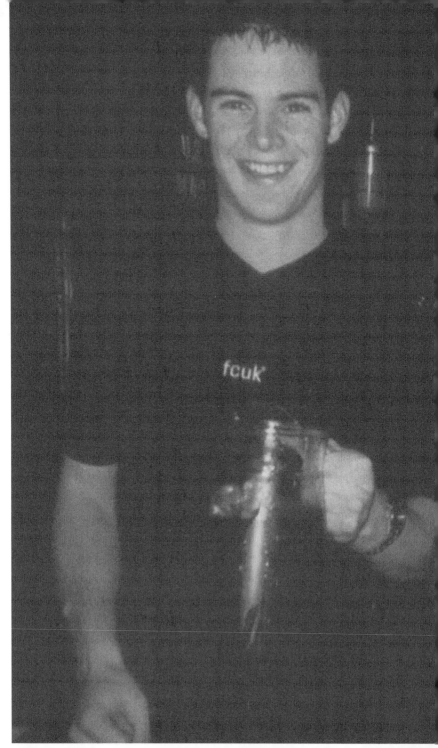

Chapter 11

Monday, 14th April, 2003
(Midnight)

The night passed the same as the others. Dan vomited a few times and needed to urinate frequently. He was still only passing a few drops at a time.

I had drifted off and my hand had slipped from his.

"Mam. MAM!"

"What is it, love?"

"I thought you'd gone."

I took his hand. "I'm here, I won't leave you." I kissed his hair. He slept again.

During the morning, a doctor came in and introduced himself as Dr O'Brien, a Consultant Urologist. He examined Dan and said "I'm certain that the primary site of the cancer is testicular. I think it can be treated with chemotherapy. Daniel needs specialist care, which we can't provide.

I'm trying to get a bed in Preston Hospital for him."

I was stunned. Two days earlier we had been told that Dan was terminally ill and now we were being told he could be treated.

Dr O'Brien continued "Daniel has a small cyst on his testes, which normally I'd remove, but he can do without an operation at the moment."

"When can he go to Preston?"

"Hopefully later today. The sooner the better."

I whispered to Dan, "We can do this, mate."

Adrenalin kicked in. I was almost hyper. We began packing up the clothes, toiletries, and foodstuff which had accumulated during the previous week. Dan's room resembled the student house.

I drove to the house to pick up some clothes and anything I thought we might need. I packed T-shirts and track bottoms for Dan, and his CD player, together with a few discs. When he was feeling stronger, he'd want to sit out of bed and listen to music.

Back at the hospital, Dr Horsley was waiting for me. "Preston won't take Daniel because his condition is too advanced. I'm trying to get a bed in Christie Hospital in Manchester. Is that alright?"

The Christie Hospital is one of the leading cancer centres in Europe. To quote an expression Dan often used, 'It's the dog's bollocks'.

Dr Horsley added "I have to warn you they may decide Daniel isn't suitable for chemotherapy." He showed me some test results. "His B.HCG is 501,847." (Beta human chorionic gonadotropin). In other words, Dan had over half a million tumour markers in his body.

I was like a cat on hot bricks. I badgered the staff. "Do you know when Dan will be transferred?"

"We're still waiting to hear." Every hour seemed to last twice as long.

Dan had another blood transfusion. He was still vomiting coffee grounds and his sputum was flecked with blood. His face had a greenish tinge. I was frightened if he deteriorated further he would be too ill to transfer.

Then we were told Dan couldn't be transferred until the next day.

My mam came down by train again. She spent time in the dayroom, so Dan wouldn't see how upset she was.

During the evening, I went to the car and phoned David Cole's mum, Maureen. I broke down, "You're the only one who knows what I'm going through. Dan's got cancer."

"No, no."

"He's going to Christie's tomorrow."

I explained quickly. Maureen said "Make sure Dan is on the Young Oncology Unit. It's specifically for his age, and he needs to see Dr Wilkinson. He's the best – he treated David. I'll phone the unit and tell them we know you. Oh, Anne. I can't believe this is happening again." She added, "I'm going to Christie's on Wednesday to collect a bag David left last time he had treatment. I'll see you then. Give Dan our love."

Dan was restless later that night. "My back's aching." I gently massaged his lower back. We weren't aware then that he had a tumour on the psoas muscle (the major muscle which links the spine and hips).

* * *

Edge Hill rugby team.

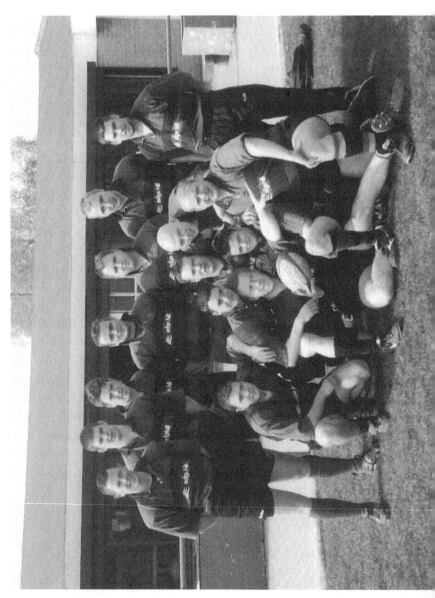

Chapter 12

Tuesday, 15th April, 2003

During the early hours Dan had stomach pains and needed the toilet. I wheeled the commode around to the bed and George and I lifted him under his arms and held him upright.

I said "You'll have to move your foot a bit, mate – I can't lock the wheel."

But Dan was unable to move his foot. He was losing the use of his limbs. We supported him while he used the commode and I cleaned him, but we couldn't get him back on the bed. I rang for a nurse. It took three of us to lift him and put him into bed. I was in pieces seeing my lad in such a state.

We waited impatiently for news of the transfer to Christie Hospital. A nurse told us Dan had to have another gastroscopy. I shook my head. "No. He's not having that again. Not after last time."

"He must have it or he can't be transferred."

When Dan realised what was being said he somehow found the energy to shout, "Mam, don't let them do that to me."

The nurse promised Dan he would be

sedated, which he was. He was not as distressed the second time.

Finally, we got the go-ahead for the transfer.

Dan's feet hung over the edge of the trolley as he was transferred from his bed. The paramedic joked with him, saying, "They make 'em long where you come from!"

I accompanied Dan in the ambulance with the paramedic and a nurse. We travelled the forty miles along the motorway in record time: lights flashing and sirens blaring. Dan woke up as the ambulance came to a halt outside the Young Oncology Unit.

I said "You've missed the blues and twos mate!"

Mike and Sam followed in their own car. He told me later, "We lost you at the first roundabout."

George had a longstanding appointment at our local hospital that day and we had decided he should keep it. Bob Jones drove him to Barrow, then to Christie's.

Dan was taken to a single, en-suite room which opened on to a lovely courtyard garden. While I dealt with the form filling, a team of nurses were looking after him. A doctor queried Dan's urine output. He said "I think there's a blockage. I want to insert a catheter to make him more comfortable."

I asked Dan "Shall I wait outside?" "NO! Stay with me."

I held his hand while the doctor inserted the catheter. "Mam, they're torturing me! Make them stop."

Within moments his urine was flowing. The doctor was pleased; it indicated that Dan's kidneys were functioning well. A blood transfusion was set up and he was put on oxygen. The mask irritated him and he kept taking it off.

The staff explained every procedure and involved us. One asked "Is it Daniel, Danny, or Dan?"

"It's Dan."

A young nurse said, "Look at his eyelashes, I wish mine were that long. He's gorgeous." Of course, I agreed with her.

Later in the evening, a nurse said, "I'll take you to the parents' accommodation and you can get settled in."

"I'm staying with Dan."

"No, you're not. You need to sleep. We'll look after him." I tried to state my case but it was futile. She assured me they would phone our room if Dan needed me.

She took us to Vicky's House, an accommodation wing which had been financed by a family whose daughter had been treated there. The wing comprised of a large lounge, kitchen, dining room and en-suite bedrooms. I have paid to stay in hotels which were not as welcoming.

At shift changeover time, a young male nurse, Damian Lacy, took over. He was friendly and asked me about Dan's lifestyle and hobbies. I reluctantly left at 11pm. Damian promised "I'll ring you if Dan needs you."

After making do with quick showers in the student house and Ormskirk Hospital, it was sheer bliss to soak in a bath! The previous days had been a roller-coaster of emotions and I was exhausted and struggling to take everything in. But I felt a bit calmer knowing Dan was being looked after.

* * *

Dan and me in September 2000

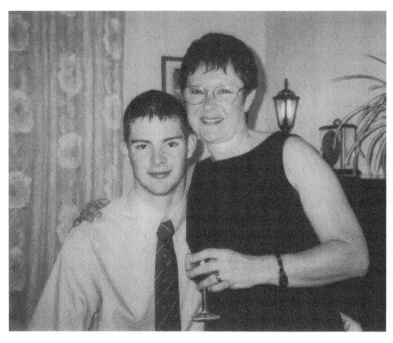

Chapter 13

Wednesday, 16th April, 2003

I woke at 7am. I had slept for nearly eight hours! I quickly washed and dressed and went to Dan's room. He had just vomited coffee grounds into the the oxygen mask and the nurses were cleaning him up.

"You've done your party piece, then," I said.

Dan was incontinent by this time. I helped the nurses give him a bed bath and change the sheets.

One of them said "I can't believe what you've done for the last week and what it took two of us to do last night." From then on, Dan received one-to-one care.

The weather was beautiful and Dan's door was open into the courtyard.

During the morning, Dr Wilkinson and his team assessed Dan. He picked up Dan's right hand and asked him to grip, which he did. He did the same with the left hand but Dan didn't respond.

Dr Wilkinson said "Push your feet against me." There was no movement from his left foot.

We met later in Dr Wilkinson's office. He said "Dan has choriocarcinoma. It's a very rare, very aggressive type of testicular cancer. I'm not pulling any punches, he's a very poorly lad. We're talking 50/50. If we can get him through the next two weeks, we're in with a chance. The cancer cells can double in 48 hours, that's how aggressive it is."

My mind refused to accept there was a fifty per cent chance that Dan would not survive.

Dr Wilkinson explained the risks of chemotherapy and told us the final decision was ours. I said "We don't have a choice, do we?"

"Yes. You do."

Without chemotherapy, Dan had no chance at all. With it, he had a slim chance. He would have it.

The first cycle of chemotherapy would commence that afternoon. But before that, a Hickman line had to be inserted. Dr Wilkinson continued "I will attempt resuscitation if Dan suffers cardiac failure."

He told us that Dan's high level of fitness had masked the symptoms. I was surprised at that, and then angry. If he was a couch potato and I'd fed him rubbish, we might have known earlier that he was ill.

Dan was drifting when we went back to his room. I explained about the Hickman line and chemotherapy. I knew he was frightened. I held his hand.

"Shall I put a CD on?"

He nodded.

"Oasis?"

Another nod.

He listened to *(What's The Story) Morning Glory?*

When Maureen Cole arrived we sat in the recreation area of the unit for a few minutes. There was a pool table, large screen TV, DVD player, music and art facilities – everything to make young cancer patients feel like normal teenagers. Maureen spoke to Dan from his doorway, and he lifted his hand slightly in greeting.

Sam drove back to Sussex at lunchtime as their little boy, Edward, was being looked after by Sam's parents.

Mike stayed to support us. He went food shopping and pressured me to eat; I managed a sandwich. He also researched the chemotherapy treatment online. It was like a foreign language to me.

I helped the nurses give Dan another bed bath.

A radiologist explained the Hickman line procedure to us. The line would be inserted through Dan's jugular vein. The procedure carried risks because of the damage to Dan's lungs caused by the tumours. My hand shook as I signed the consent form; Dan was unable to write.

The wait outside the operating theatre was agonising. A lady started talking to me, her daughter was being treated on the unit too. I just wanted her to shut up and leave me alone.

Eventually, Dan was wheeled out. The procedure had gone well. Back in Dan's room, the chemotherapy drug Etoposide was set up.

Early in the evening Dan became agitated. He cried out.

I asked "What is it, love? Are you in pain?"

"AM I IN PAIN? My head. That's the pain."

The nurse paged a doctor. I held Dan's right hand and told him to squeeze my hand. He gripped tightly, squashing my fingers on top of each other.

"How's that for a squeeze then?"

My hand was bruised for several days afterwards.

Mike bathed Dan's face in an attempt to calm him. The nurse apologised; the doctor was dealing with an emergency and she couldn't give treatment without her consent. Dan was crying and shouting. I tried unsuccessfully to soothe him.

"The doctor's on her way."

"Where's she coming from? Outer Mongolia?"

My lad still had his spark.

The doctor arrived and authorised a morphine injection. The nurse injected Dan in his buttock. "Fucking hell!"

I gasped "Daniel!"

The nurse said "Don't worry. It's not the first time someone's swore at me."

Dan calmed as the painkiller took effect.

"I'm very sorry nurse, for swearing at you."

"That's alright Dan. I know you didn't mean it."

He was critically ill and in pain, but my

son was still a gentleman.

The evening passed quietly. Nurses checked on Dan every few minutes. George sat with him while I sat outside his door in the evening sun. Then we swapped places; as I walked past the bed I knocked Dan's foot.

"Sorry, sweetheart."

He hadn't flinched. He hadn't felt anything.

* * *

Dan, Dave Barker and David Cole

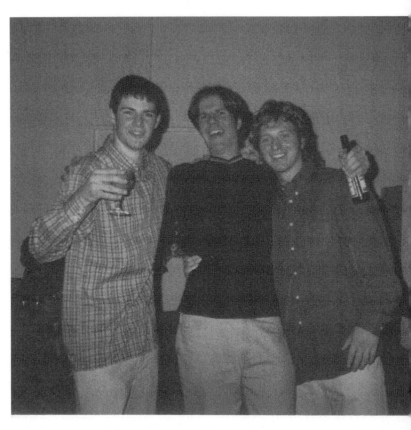

Chapter 14

Thursday, 17th April, 2003

I was dimly aware of the phone ringing. I wasn't sure where I was for a few seconds. Damian said "Dan is distressed. You need to come."

It was 2am. Still in my pyjamas, I ran down the corridor to Dan's room. George followed me, pulling his clothes on. I thought perhaps Dan was upset and had asked for me. Nothing prepared me for what I saw. Dan was propped upright on pillows. His eyes had rolled up. I think there were eight medical staff around him. Damian told me Dan was suffering respiratory failure. I took hold of Dan's hand and tried to reassure him.

"It's OK, darling. I'm here. You'll be alright."

Someone said Dan was being taken to the operating theatre for resuscitation.

I ran to our room to get dressed and woke Mike up on the way.

The team pushed Dan's bed quickly through the corridors. One nurse went in front opening the doors, two guided the bed and another supported the oxygen tank. Mike pushed the drip stand, I carried the urine bag and George had all the paperwork. We said afterwards it was like a scene from *Casualty*.

We had to wait in the nurses' kitchen near the theatre while Dan was treated. My stomach was churning. What was happening? When we were called into the theatre, Dan was sedated and attached to a ventilator. There were so many tubes and wires. A foil blanket covered him. I sat next to him and held his hand under the blanket.

Sister Pam Morrison, Clinical Resuscitation Nurse, introduced herself. She was the most compassionate, caring person. She explained every procedure that was being done to help Dan and showed me how to read the monitor. Dan's heart rate had risen to 170 – it should have been approximately 100. Pam introduced Dr Grady, an anaesthetist. I wondered why she was there? Dan wasn't having an operation. They explained it was to treat his blood gas levels.

The plan was for Dan to be transferred to an Intensive Care Unit in another hospital, as Christie's didn't have a bed for him. The staff were phoning local hospitals to check bed availability while we sat there.

We had to leave the theatre while Dan had chest x-rays taken. I went to the cloakroom. I thought If Dan opens his eyes he'll think 'Mam looks rough'. I quickly pencilled in my eyebrows.

I saw the x-rays later. Dan's lungs resembled pale grey, swirly marble.

For a couple of minutes his levels were stable, then his blood pressure dropped to 90/40.

I held Dan's hand and murmured to him. I asked Pam, "Does he know I'm here?"

"I think so. It's thought that the

hearing sense remains acute. Just keep talking to him."

She was about to freshen Dan up. "Would you like to do it?"

"Please."

I gently wiped his face, then cleaned his ears with cotton buds.

"Dan Logan, you could grow potatoes in your ears. You're a disgrace."

I smeared ointment on his eyelids to

prevent them from drying, and applied lip balm.

At 6am we had to leave the theatre while

a suction line was inserted to clear Dan's chest.

We waited in the kitchen again. The sun was coming up. I stood by the window and prayed to a god I don't believe in.

When we were called back in I sat by the head of the bed touching Dan's shoulder, while George held his hand.

Dan's levels dropped again.

"Hang on Dan. Don't leave me. You know I'm no good without you." Tears poured down my face. "Hang on, son."

Pam was emotional too. She had been on-call that night and had been with Dan since 3am. Her shift finished at 8am but she refused to leave, saying "I'm staying with Dan."

She asked if she could contact any family members. I shook my head. My parents were in their seventies and lived 120 miles away. I didn't want them to drive to Manchester.

Soon after 8am Dr Wilkinson arrived. He said "A bed is available at Wythenshawe Hospital. Dan can be transferred as soon as he's stable. I've arranged that he can still have chemotherapy in the Intensive Care Unit. But I have to be honest and tell you that he may not survive the journey."

I was beyond tears.

Dr David Tansey, a Consultant Anaesthetist, arrived from Wythenshawe Hospital. He brought a portable ventilator, which would be used for the ambulance transfer.

A nurse brought us tea and toast. I welcomed the tea but couldn't attempt to eat.

Dan's levels stabilised at about 10am and remained fairly constant. The decision was made to transfer him as soon as possible. Pam and Dr Tansey were to accompany him. I begged to go with them but there wasn't enough room in the ambulance. Mike, George and I were being taken by taxi.

I kissed Dan. "I'll see you soon, mate. I love you."

I stared blankly out of the taxi as we were driven across Manchester. I was traumatised.

We'd been told to go to the waiting room of the Critical Care Unit. George and Mike sat. I paced. Other people were waiting, but nurses were coming for them

– why was no one coming for us?

Pam came in through a side door. I rushed to her. She said "He's here and he's stable."

We hugged. I couldn't thank her enough

for everything she'd done. She said "Let me know how he is." The time was 11.50am.

We waited again. A doctor came in through the same side door and asked for Daniel Logan's family. I stood up. He said "We're working on Daniel at the moment. I'll let you know how he is as soon as I can."

What seemed like hours later but was actually about fifteen minutes, he came back and ushered us into the small side room. He introduced his colleague. I can't remember either of their names. We sat down. He said, "We were working on Daniel and something terrible happened. Daniel's heart stopped. We couldn't start it again. We tried everything. I am very, very sorry."

I fell forward, howling, "NO. NO."

George was stunned. Mike was holding his head, crying.

I gulped "Can I see him?"

"Of course. We'll disconnect the machines first."

"What time did it happen?"

"A couple of minutes ago. 12.25."

The doctor came back for us. I don't know how I walked down the corridor and through the long ward, but somehow I put one foot in front of the other. Dan was in a bay at the end of the ward. The doctor said "You can stay as long as you want. A nurse will be outside if you need her."

He pulled the curtains back.

Dan's head was turned slightly to one side. He looked as if he was asleep. I threw myself on him.

"DAN. Come back. Please come back," I sobbed.

George tried to calm me. I shook him off. I sank down on a plastic chair that someone had brought in. I clutched Dan's hand and stroked his face.

"Your nose is cold, mate."

I talked to him and touched him. My tears fell on him.

I stood up abruptly. I knew if I didn't leave at that moment I would have to be dragged out at midnight. I asked the nurse "What will happen now?"

"We'll take Daniel to the morgue."

I started crying again. What was she talking about? The words 'Daniel' and 'morgue' didn't belong in the same sentence.

She continued "We'll inform the coroner, but because it's Good Friday tomorrow, nothing will be done until Tuesday."

I kissed Dan again and walked away. I felt as though everything was in slow motion as we walked back through the ward, past the nurses' station. They stood with their heads down. I stumbled a few steps further, then turned and went back.

"You'll look after him, won't you? Because he doesn't know anyone in Manchester."

A young male nurse replied, "We'll look after him. I promise."

A taxi took us back to Christie's. The staff had been informed. They offered their help in any way, and told us we could stay in the accommodation wing as long as we wanted. We decided to go home the next day. There was nothing we could do and another family might need the room we were occupying.

I phoned my parents. They were devastated, it was impossible to take in. I phoned Jackie Jones and asked if she could come to Christie's.

I was sat on the bed crying when Jackie and Bob arrived. Jackie sat with her arms around me. I was shivering with shock. I pulled on one of Dan's tops, a grey, V-neck

Nike sweatshirt.

Jackie asked "Would you like some fresh air?"

I nodded and we walked slowly, me leaning on her, to the gardens of the main hospital. We sat on a bench. Patients and visitors were strolling around enjoying the warm Spring weather.

My son was dead.

How could the sun be shining? I was on the outside, looking in.

Back in our room, I phoned a couple of friends to break the news. They were distraught, while I was strangely calm.

Early evening, Mike and Bob went for takeaway pizza. We hadn't eaten for twenty-four hours. I didn't want to eat ever again. We found a bottle of wine in a bag which we'd brought from Ormskirk. Mike made a toast and we raised a glass to Dan.

Again, I was outside looking in.

Jackie asked "What are you planning to do with Dan's things at the student house? Would you like me to help you pack them tomorrow? It might be easier than coming back at a later date to do it."

I gratefully accepted her offer of help. We

made arrangements for the following day and they left.

I was frightened to go to bed that night. I knew, in the dark and quiet, that I would have to face the truth.

The truth that my lovely, funny, caring, handsome boy was dead.

The person who made my life worth living was dead.

I expected to be awake for hours, but shock and exhaustion knocked me out.

* * *

"Has the 'berry run out of beer?"

I was surprised to see Dan back home at 10.30pm on Christmas Eve, 2002.

"Oh very funny. The lads are all loved- up, so I thought I'd have a drink with you." The three of us had a drink together, then George went to bed.

Dan and I shared a bottle of wine and sat talking till 2am. It was as if we knew…

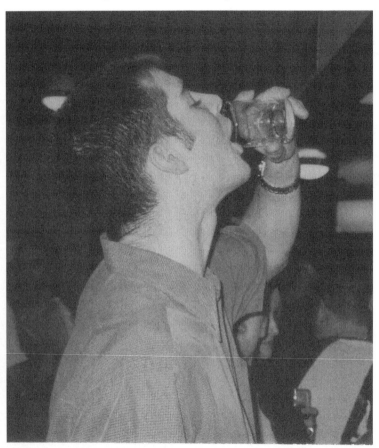

Chapter 15

Friday, 18th April, 2003

I woke and looked around the room. I didn't dream it. It happened. Dan's not here.

I was numb.

George and I were in the kitchen when Richard Cotton, a senior nurse, came in. He said "I'm really sorry to hear about Dan. It's terrible. I am sorry for your loss. I've heard from the coroner's office and I'm afraid there'll have to be a post-mortem."

That there would be a post-mortem had never occurred to me. I was horrified at the thought of Dan being cut open and I broke down sobbing.

"Why? Why do they need to do that? They know he had cancer."

"Because he was only 22 and his illness happened so quickly."

Bob arrived to take us to their home. Jonesy and I hugged and cried. He had lost his best friend.

Helen and Mark were in the student house when Jackie and I arrived. We stood with our arms around each other, crying. Jackie and I made a start on packing Dan's belongings – clothes, books, CDs, university work, rugby kits, TV and video recorder. I took the posters down from the wall and rolled them neatly. I was surprisingly calm until I came across his ticket to the Graduation Ball in his desk. Dan had planned to wear a kilt for that celebration; he loved looking smart. I leaned against the window frame and sobbed.

Dan's friends began arriving at the house. They were disbelieving. We hugged. The girls cried on each others' shoulders. Tea was made.

Once more, I was on autopilot. In my head I had already started making plans for Dan's funeral. There was nothing else I could do for him. I asked Jonesy, Sion, and Christan to be bearers – they were honoured. Christan was struggling to walk, his leg was in plaster following an operation. He said "I'll do it somehow."

I said "Will you ask three other mates? You know them better than I do." They said straightaway "Dom, Stuart and Ben."

They were tall men, apart from Jonesy, who's about 5ft 8. The lads wound him up, telling him he'd have to stretch his arms up to carry Dan.

"You know what Logan would say,

"Effin' hell, Jonesy, I'm lop-sided!" he replied. We laughed amidst the tears.

Christan said "Can you remember when he put his head through the window?"

They all sniggered then stopped, remembering I was there. "You may as well tell me now." I said.

During a houseparty Dan had tripped and gone head first through the single glazed window in the lounge. My first thought was "He could've cut his throat." He'd called a glazier the next day who'd charged him £100 for the glass and installation. The glass had to be trimmed to size and the glazier had taken the remaining piece away with him. Apparently Dan had been fuming, "That glass was mine, I've paid for it." I'm not sure what he intended to do with it . . .

I went back to the funeral plans, "Should Dan wear a suit or rugby kit?"

Christan answered "He loved getting dressed up didn't he."

"Yeah, suit, shirt, and tie. That's it."

Dan's student life was packed up. Everyone helped to carry the boxes and holdalls downstairs. I sobbed as I carried an armful of Dan's shirts. We loaded up three cars. I was travelling with Jackie, Bob was driving Dan's car, and George was driving mine (which he'd driven to Ormskirk the previous week).

Dan's friends stood on the pavement.

None of us spoke.

I was crying.

We arrived in Barrow early in the evening. The avenue was deserted. I walked into our home: the home I had left exactly two weeks ago, with an overnight bag, thinking I was going to give my son some TLC because he had a virus.

Everything looked the same.

But nothing would ever be the same again.

* * *

The broken window, and the remorseful Dan!

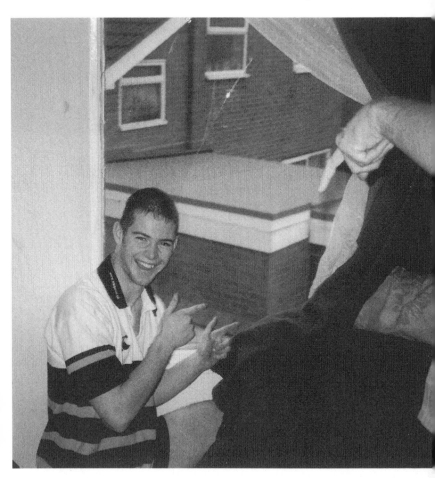

Chapter 16

Dan's post mortem revealed:

- Multiple nodules throughout the brain parenchyma and the brain surface.
- Both lungs were studded with brown tumour nodules.
- The left ventricle contained a grey/brown mass, approximately 3.5cm.
- The stomach contained multiple, brown, mucosal lesions.
- In part of the duodenum was a 2cm tumour.
- The small intestine had a 2.5cm tumour.
- Multiple tumour nodules in the small bowel mesentery.
- A 12cm retroperitineal tumour mass anterior to the psoas muscle at the beginning of the large intestine.
- The liver contained numerous haemorrhagic tumour masses.
- Both kidneys contained multiple brown tumour deposits.

David Cole and his family visited us at home two days after Dan's death. David had endured several major surgeries and countless cyles of chemotherapy; he was terminally ill. We stood with our arms around each other and he said quietly, "Be glad he went as he did, Anne. I wouldn't want anyone to go through this."

David's words comforted me that day

and they still do. Sadly, he died on 23rd July 2003, three months after Dan. I believe those fabulous young men are together.

Dan and David have a conference suite named after them at Hoops Basketball Centre in Barrow.

How Dare You

Anne Logan Huxtable 2014

You grew unexpectedly. Silently.
Devious and cruel; you hid the signs.
He didn't know you existed.
How dare you.

Your filthy cells multiplied.
You made him cough.
You made him bleed.
You caused him pain.
How dare you.

He fought but you were too strong.
You took his dreams.
His ambitions.
You took his chance for a child to call him Dad.
Then you took him.
How dare you.

You took my reason for living, that day.
You took my future.
You took my son.
How dare you.

Chapter 17

Tuesday, 29th April, 2003
(1.30pm)

The cortege drove slowly through the streets towards Thorncliffe Crematorium.

Every time we halted at a junction, I thought, *That's my Dan in front. It can't be. In that box. You know it is.*

I was waiting for someone to tell me there had been a mistake and Dan was still here.

Cars, minibuses, and coaches were parked bumper-to-bumper along the hill leading to the cemetery gates.

I stood on the path, staring blankly. I was suited and booted, the same as Dan.

The undertakers assisted the bearers, Dan Jones, Christan Upton, Sion Williams, Dom and Stuart Carter, and Ben Moss, to lift Dan onto their shoulders. They stumbled as they reached the doorway; our floral tribute of a rugby ball wobbled. I murmured "Don't drop him."

The crematorium was packed, people stood at the back, the foyer was full and many more stood outside.

We had chosen one of Dan's favourite songs, *Babylon* by David Gray, to start the ceremony.

George and I gripped each other's hands and followed Dan inside.

The secular ceremony was taken by Terry Bartlett, who had been recommended by David Caine, the funeral director. He welcomed everyone, then introduced George's brother-in-law, Tim Fisher. Tim read out my personal tribute to Dan, which included a story of he and I going to Murrayfield to see Scotland v The All Blacks. Everyone sang Flower of Scotland, a rugby anthem that Dan loved.

Terry introduced Paul Woodward, Dan's rugby coach from Liverpool St Helens. Paul put down his prepared speech and spoke from the heart. He said what a great person Dan was and how easily he had fitted in the with team. He told of how keen Dan was to progress at rugby and that even at a cold, windy training session, he would make them all laugh.

He said "If Dan's listening now, he'll be thinking, 'Stop waffling Woody.'"

Terry then read the poem Do not stand at my grave and weep.

A joint tribute from George and myself was next, followed by a couple of minutes reflective silence.

I had requested that everyone listen to Wonderwall by Oasis, Dan's psyching-up song. The next track on the disc, Don't Look Back in Anger, began; that was our cue to leave. I refused to get up from my seat. I knew once I walked out, it really was final. If I stayed I was still with Dan.

Despite being pulled and cajoled, I wouldn't move.

Eventually, I stood up. David Caine ushered me outside. I leaned against the railings, gasping for breath. He said "Would you like to speak to a few people, then see how you feel?" I nodded.

About three hundred people paid their respects in the receiving line: Dan's former schoolmates and teachers, basketball players, Vickers, Edge Hill and Liverpool St. Helens rugby communities, mates and staff from Edge Hill University, neighbours, my friends and work colleagues, plus those of George.

Most were still in tears; big strapping rugby players not afraid to show their emotions. I was hugely comforted by their words about Dan.

Dan's wake was held at Vickers Rugby Club, (now Hawcoat Park). I asked a couple of his mates, "Do you think he would've liked the ceremony?"

"He would've loved it."

I wandered around, speaking to people, almost as if I was the hostess at a party. It was surreal. What am I doing here?

As the beers went down, the atmosphere became more relaxed, and the rugby teams challenged each other to a drinking competition. One of my abiding memories of that day is watching Martin Sainty and Neil France as they turned in a circle, singing *'Turn around you warriors'*, as the teams belted out *Sunshine Mountain*.

At one point, the Vickers lads formed a huddle. Someone shouted "Anne, come on."

I shook my head, "No. I can't."

George said "Go on. Dan isn't here, they want you in his place."

I joined in with them, bonding.

The evening turned into a rugby party.

Dan would have been in his element!

A few weeks earlier, I had asked Dan "Are you coming home at the weekend to catch up with the lads?" (Which also meant that I wanted to see him).

He replied "No, the Vickers lads have forgotten about me now."

Dan, you were so wrong.

They loved you and respected you.

No one could have had a better farewell.

* * *

It was raining heavily as Christan and Jonesy left Dan's wake late on Tuesday night. They were brimming with emotion and alcohol and collapsed on the back seats of a parked car at the bottom of Vickers' club driveway. What they thought was a taxi was, in fact, a police car.

Phil Bygrave thought they'd been arrested and started shouting and banging on the windows. The police driver said "Right lads, that's it. We would've given you a lift but you've spoilt it for yourselves. Get out."

Christan told me "It's the first time I've ever been thrown OUT of a police car!"

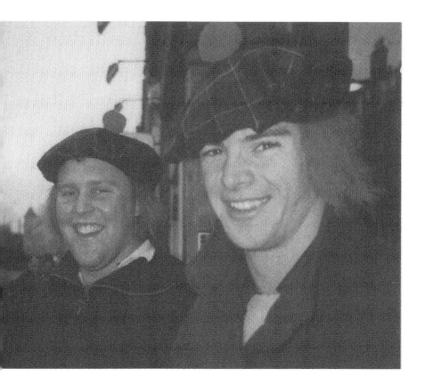

Chapter 18

Events

Dan was awarded a BSc 2.2 Degree in Sports Science and Education Studies from Edge Hill University. He had handed in his dissertation and had one exam left to sit. We couldn't contemplate attending the graduation ceremony, it was only a few weeks after Dan's death. The staff kindly organised a small, informal ceremony and buffet in September. Dan's mates were invited too.

Dan's tutors spoke highly of him; he was conscientious and well-liked. The terrace outside the Sports Institute had been carpeted with flowers on the first day back after the Easter holidays.

I broke down when the Vice- Chancellor handed me Dan's degree.

"I feel a fraud. Dan should be collecting this, not me. I haven't earned it." It was an emotional, uplifting afternoon, followed by celebratory drinks with the usual suspects in a local pub, then dinner with the Jones family at their home.

* * *

Donations from Dan's funeral amounted to £4,174, which we presented to the Young Oncology Unit at Christie Hospital.

* * *

Dan Jones completed two treks in Dan's memory; Mount Kilimanjaro and Everest Base Camp. He raised over £10,000 for the Young Oncology Unit.

* * *

Thorns Basketball Club and Edge Hill University also held fundraising events.

* * *

Vickers Rugby Club (overleaf) held a fabulous gala day and evening disco the following summer. The Vickers and Edge Hill teams played for the Dan Logan Memorial Trophy. £1,417 was donated to Christie Hospital.

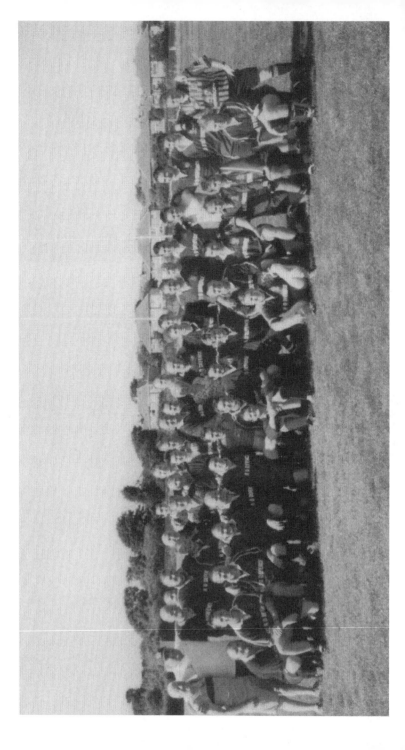

Aftermath

It has been said that,
'Time heals all wounds.'
I do not agree. The wounds remain.
In time, the mind, protecting its sanity
covers them with scar tissue,
and the pain lessens.
But it is never gone.

Rose Kennedy

Two days after the Vickers Gala Day, in August 2004, George died suddenly from a heart attack.

In the space of sixteen months I had lost my only child and my husband.

George had been my rock after Dan died. I didn't grieve for him for a long time

– I was angry with him because he'd left me, plus I had nothing left to give; I was exhausted emotionally and mentally.

I spiralled into the black hole.

I ate just enough to get by on; my weight dropped to seven and a half stones. Many evenings I drank myself into a stupor, waking up on the sofa at 3 or 4am and then staggering to bed. I'm not proud of that; but the pain was blocked out for a

few hours.

I felt an overwhelming sense of guilt. Why hadn't I known that Dan was ill?

What kind of mother was I? It had been my job to protect him.

Alongside the guilt was anger. Anger at filthy, evil cancer. Anger that there are so many bad people in the world – why were they still here when Dan wasn't? Why was my wonderful son's future taken from him?

When the phone rang, or someone knocked on the door, for a split second, I would think That's Dan, followed by the gut-wrenching knowledge that it would never be Dan.

The loss of a child is not something which can be 'got over' or 'moved on' from. The loss is all-encompassing.

I wanted my life to be over.

But I knew Dan would be mad if I ended it. That would be my choice.

Epilogue

Our family had a reason to smile again when Mike and Sam's second son, Christopher Daniel, was born in the summer of 2005.

Earlier that year, my lovely,

supportive friend Brenda suggested that she and I had a week in the sun. In the Shamrock Bar in Gran Canaria, in May 2005, I met the man who would change my life.

'Tipperary Sean' was singing regional songs and someone chose Flower of

Scotland.

I was ambushed by emotion, tears poured down my face. Bren comforted me. She said afterwards "I didn't know whether to push you outside or buy you a double gin!"

Later that evening, after some banter, we joined three middle-aged men at their table. There was an instant, mutual attraction between myself and David, a tall, broad Welshman. He asked "Are you OK? I saw you crying."

"Flower of Scotland was my son's funeral song. He died two years ago."

Most men would've done a four-minute

mile. But David didn't. He asked about Dan. At that time, I didn't talk about Dan to people who hadn't known him, but David was easy to talk to. We talked for hours, long after our friends had left, then he ushered me to a taxi.

We met 'accidentally' the night Liverpool won the European Champion- ship. We had a few drinks and sat on a bench talking until the early hours. On the last night of our holidays we went out for a drink; we both knew then it was more than a holiday romance. That evening, David said to me, "I'm not going to lose you now that I've found you."

We spoke several times a day the following week, then David came to Barrow for the weekend.

The following month, I went to Cardiff for two weeks. I knew that was where I wanted to be. I also knew I would regret it if I didn't grab the chance of starting a new life. Despite warnings of 'You don't know him properly', and 'Are you sure you know what you're doing?' I moved to Cardiff in October that year, along with Jakesie Cat! I told David at the beginning of our relationship, "We come as a unit; me, Dan, and the cat." He wasn't overly keen on the cat...

David is the most genuine, loving person. He looks after me and supports me in everything I do.

And he makes me laugh. David only knows the person I am now, he didn't know the me 'before'. Because I'm not the same person I was when Dan was alive. I hope I'm more compassionate and caring, but I now operate a 'zero tolerance' policy.

On 8th September 2007 David and I were married. We shared a lovely day with close family and friends. If anyone had told me two years previously that I could have a day like that, I would've said they were mad. We always say Dan brought us together.

A few months after relocating I heard of The Compassionate Friends, a charity which supports bereaved parents after the loss of a child/children. While using the online support forum I met two mothers from my area and we've become good friends.

Later that year, I read an article about the charity Teenage Cancer Trust and the unit which was under construction at the University Hospital of Wales, in Cardiff. The units provide specialist treatment, in an age-appropriate environment, for young people aged 13-24 who have cancer. I joined the local fundraising committee; and independently raised thousands of pounds by organising sponsored walks, coffee mornings, a choir concert, and a firewalk. (I've walked over burning coals for you, Dan!).

But I needed to do more.

I'm not, nor have ever been, religious.

But I do believe in an afterlife, that a person's spirit lives on when the physical body has died. So I visited a medium in 2009. She described Dan physically and said "He has beautiful eyes."

She told me Dan was showing her a pen, an old-fashioned quill, and said, "He wants you to write."

Well, what am I supposed to write about? I wondered.

In 2012 I visited another medium. During the meeting he said, "I can see traditional old rooms. Have you stayed in a cottage or hotel with open fires and beams?"

"No," I replied.

"Are you planning to stay somewhere like that?"

I wasn't: I prefer modern accommodation. Anyone who knows me knows I'm a townie! The medium continued "You enjoy writing, don't you? Your son wants you to write his story. Not for fame or celebrity, but because people will be interested in what you have to say. He's saying 'Get it out there.'"

I was taken aback to put it mildly – English was my best subject at school but I couldn't write a book!

Soon after I moved to Cardiff, I began seeing a holistic therapist and reflexologist, Fiona Akpinar, a wise, serene lady who has since become a good friend. Dan gave me messages through her: once he showed her a muddy rugby kit soaking in a bucket in the kitchen of our old home; he and I were laughing. After another treatment, Fiona said "Dan showed me a pen. He said it's special and you'll know what it is."

The pen in question was given to me by Dan's friends at his degree presentation – it was his Edge Hill Graduate 2003 pen.

The idea of writing about Dan grew stronger, but how would I do it? I had a lot to learn before I could begin.

I enrolled on a creative writing course run by the talented children's author Jon Blake.

Everything I learned on the course would go on to help me when I started writing about Dan. I felt a bit out of my depth at the first session – the other students were teachers and journalists – but everyone was friendly. I went on to complete a short story course and writing for children course and became a member of local writing group, Parkwriters.

In May 2015 Jon organised a weekend writing retreat at Cilwych Farm Cottages, near Bwlch in the stunning Brecon Becons. I gasped as I walked into the beautiful, converted farm buildings, complete with open fireplaces and beams!

Jon held morning and afternoon group sessions to enable us to discuss our writing and receive feedback. I was very apprehensive; I was away from David and completely out of my comfort zone. I was baring my soul to people I'd never met, but my fellow writers were supportive and encouraging. I asked "Am I on the right track before I go any further?" They assured me I was and offered constructive advice over a few glasses of wine!

I continued writing and researching throughout the summer. I already had copies of Dan's medical records from Ormskirk, Christie and Wythenshaw Hospitals and also a copy of his post mortem report. While writing, I relived those awful days when Dan was ill; it was a harrowing and painful time.

Jon organised a second retreat in September 2015 at the same beautiful location.

I had decided it would be too hard to write about Dan's last day while I was there, but on Sunday morning a favourite saying of Dan's came into my mind: 'Just do it'. I was spurred on: by mid-afternoon I had completed the first draft of Dan's Story.

I was too emotional to read my work aloud; (thank you Jan Farrell for reading it on my behalf). I could never have envisaged the reaction of my fellow writers. Parents and non-parents, male and female, were all in tears. Mario walked across the lounge and kissed my cheek. He couldn't speak. They empathised with my loss and urged me to continue writing, with the aim of Dan's Story being published. We shared a bond that day, even though some of them had been strangers two days earlier.

My sincere thanks go to Jon, Mario, Li, Kath, Sarah, Jan, Sara, and Rachel for your support and kindness.

* * *

Thirteen years later, I'm still stunned by the speed at which cancer took Dan. No words can describe the pain of losing my only child. I've learned to live alongside the constant ache; it's a part of who I am.

I still shy away like a hermit at times, still fall into the 'black hole', but I owe it to Dan to live my life to the best of my ability. I share good times with my lovely David, we enjoy concerts and holidays, but there's always a part of my life missing.

The part where my son should be.

I'm in touch with Dan's mates from Barrow and Edge Hill, some now live abroad; I'm happy they are living their lives, but it's bittersweet when I hear of a wedding or a new baby. I think, YOU should be here, doing this.

* * *

Dan still influences me. When I need advice I think, What would Dan say? and I know what his response would be – it's usually, Let it go, Mam!

So after sixteen months of blood, sweat and tears, your story is 'out there', son.

Dan, I hope I've made you proud.

Acknowledgements

Thank you to Jon Blake for editing and guidance.

To my reading team of Fiona Akpinar, Brenda Clark, Jackie Jones, Jane Mullins, Maria Nicholas, Hayley Sainty, and Martin Sainty.

Thank you, Dr Ann Williams, for your support.

To the Parkwriters for your encouragement.

Grateful thanks to David Norrington for your advice.

Last, but not least, to my lovely David, thank you for everything.

Teenage Cancer Trust

is a charity that funds specialist units in
NHS hospitals for young cancer patients
aged 13-24, enabling them to be treated
by experts in a place designed
especially for them.

www.teenagecancertrust.org

The Compassionate Friends (UK)

is a charity dedicated to the support
of bereaved parents, siblings and
grandparents after the loss
of a child, from any cause.

Helpline: 0345 123 2304
www.tfc.co.uk

Printed in Great Britain
by Amazon